John McDillon

WEIGHT TRAINING

FOR BEGINNERS

A Complete Illustrated Guide to Strength Training at Home for Men and Women. Easy and Effective Exercises and Workouts with Free Weights to Burn Fat and Build Muscle

I am strong

I'm fit

I'll make it

My determination is firm

Table of Contents

INTRODUCTION

The goal of this program is to help you achieve a better fit, lose weight and develop the necessary fitness and cardiovascular basis you need to achieve your goals. Follow-up programs are available, and you can prepare for your next level of fitness. However, if you train with this e-book, you have to achieve two goals.

➢ Build a fitness base
➢ Lose weight

DO YOU HAVE TIME TO EXERCISE?

Do you not have enough time to exercise on your day? Too many people say, "I have to exercise, but I don't have enough time for the day." Or if you have the time, you have the energy to lie down and watch TV. Whether you're on business, working at home, working with family, or holding other post-school events, the following schedule or a version of it can help you overcome your problems.

Exercise is more than sleeping or sitting. You can use abdominal exercises to move your upper body or other upper body exercises, even if your back or abdomen is on a flat floor. Pushups are a great "lying exercise," and abdominal cramps are a little more complicated than sleeping. An hour a day is an admirable goal to improve your fitness level and overall health, but even 10-15 minutes are more effective than nothing.

Getting fit in one day is a challenge that we all have to face. Exercising after long hours at home, in the office, or on the street is difficult, but it still creates a generation of people with obesity and other preventable health problems, so Americans still have to exercise. Many people who have difficulty keeping their fitness on schedule can get their work done 15 to 20 minutes before the start of the day and 15 to 20 minutes after the end of the day. I'm going. Even if the exercise is a simple walk before breakfast and after dinner, a 15 to 20-minute walk at any of these times can help significantly burn calories that only accumulate as fat. An easy walk and some gymnastics after a meal can help increase your energy levels and help you do everything.

HERE IS THE SCHEDULE I USUALLY DO FOR BUSY DAYS WHEN A LONG DAY COMES:

- 06:00 - Get up early to do aerobic exercise such as running, cycling, or swimming for 20 to 30 minutes. When you're on the go, find the hotel pool and wake up for the day.
- 07:00 - Have breakfast for the energy of the day. (See Lean Down Food Plan)
- 08:00 - work

    - Work-eat a snack

- 12:30 - eat lunch
- 1:15 - Walk a few minutes
- 1:30 - work
- 4:00 am - Work - Eat a snack
- 6:00 - break for dinner

➤ 7:00 - PT for walking or lifting weights or for a second wind on long days

➤ 8:00 - continue working until midnight if necessary

I want to do cardio training early in the morning when I have to work 15 to 18 hours. That woke me up completely, and I am ready to take care of the day before. Next, enjoy a delicious breakfast of protein, carbohydrates, and plenty of water. Then pack midnight snacks like apples, oranges, yoghurt, and nutritional bars. It will help you become a greedy canteen at lunch in the restaurant. For lunch, a green leafy salad with red meat like chicken, fish and boiled eggs. Then take a 10-15 minute walk to maintain your afternoon metabolism. If you put away bread, pure sugar and protein foods, complex carbohydrates and fibre, your afternoon work will be much easier. After the rest of the day, take a break for a mid-sized dinner and go again if you don't have weights, no short workouts, or these facilities. But a training session or PT gives us the second wind we need to work and play with our family. I hope these tips are helpful because they are common problems we see today. Remember that something is better than anything else. Go out and go at least several times a day.

FIVE PHASES OF FITNESS (PSYCHOLOGICAL)

Below are five phases we all experience when we start a new fitness program, regardless of what level of fitness we have.

➢ Make a decision to be healthy ... this takes 3-4 seconds, but it takes about 2-3 weeks to make a habit - stays there at least long ... and build a practice well on.

➢ You doubt yourself. It is natural to ask what you are trying to do. My advice is to challenge yourself and get over it as soon as possible. Understand that self-doubt is part of the process ... Even SEAL trainees challenge themselves, but those who become SEAL overcome their doubts.

➢ Overcome the suspicion - you can do anything you can imagine. You said that to yourself now. Here mind and body connect. Used to promote education in all areas of life, including work, relationships and school. I am convinced that by training your body, your stamina and energy can exercise your spirit and build a better relationship. Things around you ...

➢ Connect with a healthy and healthy person. Now adjust your mind and body. Your example will inspire others. It plays the role of model for other heavy people. People will be excited about your new work ethic, work and play. A healthy diet is still your habit ... When you eat grumpy foods, you feel a little sick.

➤ Set your own goals and conquer. Whatever you like - run, increase your bike weight ... challenge yourself, run 10 km, lift 400 pounds ...

AN ESSENTIAL GUIDE TO STRENGTH TRAINING

Basics and programs of strength training:

The basis for successful strength training is a combination of elements that are sometimes referred to as FITT.

- ➤ Training frequency - frequency
- ➤ Training intensity - how difficult it is
- ➤ Time spent - session time
- ➤ Exercise type - which exercise
- ➤ Muscle and exercise
- ➤ Understanding the muscles and how they work is vital for strength training.
- ➤ There are two types of muscle contraction.

➢ Isometric contraction: muscles do not stretch. An example of this is pushing a wall.

➢ Isotonic contractions: The muscles become shorter and more extended. The shortening phase is called "concentric: contraction" and the extension phase is called "eccentric" contraction.

For example, the curl of the barbell arm shortens the muscles (concentric circles) when you lift the barbell and lengthens (eccentricity) when you lower it. Eccentric contractions mainly cause muscle pain.

COMMON MOVEMENT

Muscle contraction is related to joint mobility. The four most critical collective actions are flexion and extension, abduction and adduction.

➢ Flexion is the reduction of joint angles. An example is an upward movement of the arms curvature that reduces the aspect of the elbow joint.

➢ Extension is the opposite movement. Increase the edge while reducing weight.

➢ Abduction is the removal of a body part from the centre of the side body. For example, raise your legs to the side of your body.

➢ The adduction brings part of the body closer to the midline of the body.

MUSCLE GROUP

The main muscle groups that make up the human body are the abdomen, the adductors (inner thigh), the back muscles (middle back), the shoulders, the extensor muscles of the wrist, the extensor wrists, the gluteus muscles (buttocks), the flexor arm, the flexor wrist muscle, Shoulder blade fixation muscle. (Shoulder blade), flexor muscle (thigh), psoas muscle (waist), sternum (calf), pectoral muscle (chest), quadriceps femoris (front of the thigh) and trapezius muscle (upper back).

If you look closely, the main muscle groups are the arms, shoulders, chest, back, legs, buttocks, and abdomen. There are several ways to address all major muscle groups during exercise.

➢ Do a variety of activities that move your body in one session (high-intensity interval training, HIIT, Cross Fit training, etc.).

➢ You can do a body part splitting exercise that is common in conventional bodybuilding training (days focusing on the upper body, days focusing on the lower body, etc.).

➢ Concentrate on more massive exercises (squats, bench press, deadlifts, cleansing and jerking, snapping) that focus on large muscle groups.

A PERSON RESPONSIBLE, HIRED, RM

You need to know these basic terms that are used in training.

➤ A repetition is the end of an exercise. One is the chin, one is the crouch, and one is the arm curl.

➤ Set is the number of repetitions that you have selected before a break. Suppose a set of arm curls has ten repetitions.

➤ The pause interval is the time between sentences.

➤ A maximum of 1 rpm or iterations is your personal best or the maximum that you can lift once with each exercise. So the 12RM is the largest you can lift in 12 reps.

So how do you know who is responsible, how many sentences, and how much time is left? Overall, it looks like this: You and your trainer can work with the finer details.

➢ Weight training uses the most weight, the least number of iterations, and the most extended break.

➢ Hypertrophic or muscular workouts require less weight, more repetitions and less rest.

➢ Strength endurance is rebalanced, repeated and less rested.

➢ Strength training focuses on the speed of the lift, is comfortable and has long breaks.

These are general principles. Customize your sets, your staff, your breaks and your exercise types to find the perfect combination.

An example based on a theoretical personal best of 73 kg (160 pounds), a bench press exercise program looks like this according to various goals:

➢ Bench press-1RM = 160 lbs
➢ Strength: 140 lbs, 2 x 5, 180 seconds
➢ Hypertrophy: 120 lbs, 3 x 10, 60 seconds
➢ Strength endurance: 100 lbs, 3 x 15, 45 seconds
➢ Power: 90 lbs, 3 x 8, 120 seconds

One thing to keep in mind here is that for optimal results, you must have an adequate break between your strength training groups. A good rest interval is also important during strength training since each explosion must be carried out at a high burst rate to achieve maximum effectiveness. Therefore, strength and strength training should ensure that you get the rest you need between sets. It is ideal for hypertrophy and strength endurance if possible, but shorter intervals are less important.

SPEED OF EXERCISE EXECUTION

The contraction rate is the rate at which the training is carried out, which also affects the training results. Here are some general guidelines for weight training goals:

- Strength: 1-2 seconds of concentric circles and eccentricity
- Hypertrophy: 2-5 seconds of concentric circles and eccentricity
- Endurance: 1-2 seconds of concentric circles and eccentricity
- Power: concentric circles less than 1 second, eccentricity 1-2 seconds

CALCULATION OF 1RM

According to the US National Strength and Conditioning Association, the percentage of 1 rpm, the theoretical repetition distribution for maximum buoyancy, is distributed as follows, using 160 lbs 1 rpm for the bench press.

➤ 100% of 1 rpm: 160 lbs - one repetition

➤ 85% of 1 RM: £ 136 - 6 reps

➤ 67% of 1 rpm: 107 lbs - 12 reps

➤ 65% of 1 rpm: 104 lbs - 15 repetitions

➤ 60% of 1RM: £ 96 - warm-up staff

That is, one elevator is a personal best, six lifts are 85% off a personal best, 15 bins is a personal best of

1rpm at 65% of all elevators in between, and probably less...

Do not consider this an absolute reference. This is a guide and the basis for choosing the right weights for your workout.

BUILD STRENGTH

Muscle strength, size and endurance are built on the principle of overload. This requires more and more heavy loads and more overtime.

In contrast to increased muscle size (called hypertrophy), strength is not the muscle anatomy, size and composition of the muscle fibres. Still, the interaction between the neuromuscular system and the nerves and muscles is built through training and to prioritize strength, a higher weight with fewer repetitions and more extended rest periods is used.

Larger muscles usually make you stronger, but maybe less healthy than those who exercise when everyone else is the same.

The strength training includes loads in the range from 3 to 6 rpm for experienced lifters and higher loads from 1 to 3 pm, the number of sets varies depending on the program.

BUILD MUSCLE SIZE

Hypertrophy training usually emphasizes more reps with lighter weights than weight training and often results in shorter pause intervals between sets. This workout strengthens metabolic factors that increase size.

You can train more for hypertrophy, but if you're interested in bodybuilding or powerlifting, your goals should be apparent. If you need a combination of strength and hypertrophy, you need to identify a strength training program that offers a compromise. This is what most non-competitive strength coaches want.

One way in which muscles grow is through the process of micro-level damage and repair. Small tears, sometimes referred to as minor trauma, develop in the muscle fibres under load and are repaired and rebuilt when the trainer recovers. It's like a step back and two steps forward at the cellular phone level.

There is disagreement as to whether muscle fibres (cells) grow in size or whether they divide and form new cells to enlarge the muscles. At the very least, hypertrophy is due to an increase in contractile units called myofibrils and an increase in an intracellular fluid called muscle mass.

Hypertrophic training typically uses 8-12 RM iterations with a variable number of sets, but often in the range of 2 to 5.

BUILD MUSCLE ENDURANCE

Muscle endurance is trained at the top of the repeating spectrum. For example, if you do 15 to 20 iterations per set, your goal is local muscle endurance, not strength or hypertrophy. Again, this type of muscle endurance training offers some strength and hypertrophy compared to no training and can significantly improve aerobic conditioning compared to high-intensity programs. For muscle endurance training, you can use repetitions in the range of 15 to 20, and the number of sets is variable, but three is standard. However, for training skills like running, swimming, and cycling, you need to ask yourself if this is a productive use of your time.

BUILD MUSCLE STRENGTH

Electricity is time-consuming because it is the speed at which you work. If you can lift the same weight faster than your friends, you will have more strength. Strength training involves increasing the lifting speed. The concept of resistance helps with strength training in sports such as football, where strength, mass and acceleration are desired.

In strength training, you build muscle strength first and then move on to light loads that are performed at very fast or explosive contraction rates. The American College of Sports Medicine recommends a light load of 30-60% 1rpm for 2-3 minutes between sets.

Strength training, strength training or strength training form the basis for durability, strength, mass and endurance in your next activity or sport as you like.

➤ Bodybuilding, specializing in body shaping and muscle definition, especially for competitive purposes. The bloating program is the mainstream here.

➤ Sport-specific programs use exercises to support and improve the muscle movements of the sport as much as possible. One example is training a swimmer with exercises that target the shoulder, arm and back muscles to simulate underwater pulling movements. Strength, endurance, mass and strength programs are useful but very diverse for a specific sport and should be designed so that they do not affect the skills required for the sport.

➢ Weight Loss and Fitness includes exercises that offer a comprehensive training program to build muscle and reduce body fat. This includes bodybuilders who just look good on the beach.

➢ Olympic weightlifting is an individual weightlifting sport that uses only two exercises: clean jerking and tearing, although there are many training exercises. Every lift is highly specialized, technical and requires a lot of training and practice.

➢ Powerlifting competitions only require three lifts: squats, bench presses and deadlifts. Here too, strength and technology programs are the basis for powerlifting.

TRAINING FREQUENCY AND OVERTRAINING

The frequency and extent of the training depend on your goals, your experience, your age, your health, your fitness and other factors such as B. Accessibility of your equipment and time available for training. The trainer or coach needs to consider all of these factors and design a plan that fits the situation and goals.

The delicate balance of strength training is the balance between stimulation, adaptation and recovery of the muscle and nervous system. Excessive intensity, loudness, too fast frequency and overtraining syndrome can disrupt your progress. Signs of overtraining are:

➢ Persistent fatigue, poor performance

➢ Viral and bacterial infections

➢ Accidental weight loss

➢ Regular damage to the musculoskeletal system

➢ suspension or irregularity

➢ Hormonal imbalance

➢ Reduced bone density

➢ Bad sleeping and eating behavior

Training three times a week is an ideal place for beginners, while training is suitable for some twice a day for seven days. The usual recommendation for beginners is to allow at least 48 hours between weight sessions to allow recovery.

For experienced and professional trainers, training six days a week is not uncommon, but a split system (training different muscle groups on various days) is often carried out. If you feel that something is wrong, step back and get the appropriate advice.

EXERCISE TYPE

With hundreds of exercises for many muscles and muscle groups, the average beginner is not too confused to decide. Exercise variants are delivered with free weights, machines, frames and frames, body-only exercises, bands, balls and much more. Therefore, exercise types can be categorized by device type, muscle target or even fitness target. For example, aerobic or strength exercises, treadmills or lat pulldown machines.

➤ Combined exercises. Complex exercises involve multiple joints, often various large muscle groups. Examples: squats, deadlifts, seated cable cars, latitude pulldowns.

➤ Separation exercises. A single workout is a movement that involves only one joint and is usually aimed at isolated muscle groups. Examples include barbell curls for the biceps and leg extension for the quadriceps.

WHICH EXERCISE SHOULD I DO?

It depends on your goals, the equipment available, your age, your strength, your weight experience and your commitment.

Suppose you want to increase strength and muscle mass. There is general agreement that "Big 3" powerlifting lifts (squats, bench presses, deadlifts) are core lifts for building mass and strength. They are technical and maybe even dangerous, but leadership and spotters are essential because they are carried out with free weights close to their maximum. Still, it's a smooth start to understand the point and move on.

When exercising to balance body composition and strength, you should add back, abdominal, and shoulder movements to the three larger bodies to do more specific work in front of your arms. This basic strength program offers a recommended set of exercises. Most gyms have a variety of equipment to perform these exercises.

In bodybuilding, where even the smallest muscles can have significant muscle definitions, there is usually a more comprehensive range of isolated movements. Olympic weightlifting requires specific strength and technique training.

Strength training program

A training program, whether strength training or other fitness training, is a schedule for training frequency, intensity, volume and type. Weight training uses a variety of methods and techniques.

You can adjust the following variables in the strength training program. Almost unlimited combinations are possible, most of which work at a certain level, but are not always optimal.

➢ Exercise selection

➢ Weight or resistance

➢ Number of repetitions

➢ Number of sentences

➢ Movement speed

➢ Distance between sentences

➢ Interval between sessions (training days/weeks)

➢ Periodic cycle interval

HERE ARE SOME OF THE MOST GENERAL APPLICATIONS AND TECHNIQUES FOR STRENGTH TRAINING AND BODYBUILDING PROGRAMMING.

➢ Whole-body training. Exercise all major muscle groups in the session. Choose a range of elevators (probably up to 10). Make sure that all major muscle groups work out at a certain level.

➢ Partition the system. Alternative sessions for essential muscle groups. Training, for example, one session for arms, shoulders, back, then hips for legs, next meeting for the belly.

➢ Regularization can be described as a progressive or cyclical training phase over a specified period to achieve a result at a specified point in time. An example is the division of the annual program into different training modalities with different successive goals. This is common in sports-specific programs and competition formats for weight lifting. For example, maintenance out of season, fitness before the season, bloating and strength before the season, active maintenance in the season, recovery after the season.

➢ Superset. The super setting is a practice in which two opposing muscle groups are trained in quick succession to stimulate muscle growth and alternating rest in both groups. Examples include quad extension and hamstring of the hamstring and leg flexion.

➢ Compound set. The assembled collection does not change between different muscle groups, but between exercises or equipment for the same muscle group. As an example, we follow the triceps setback with a triceps pushdown. This serves to push the muscles in so far that additional motor units can be recruited.

➢ pyramid. This type of program includes a series of exercises that range from easy to challenging for the same training, or vice versa, from testing to accessible for some programs. Enter the number of records. For example, dumbbell curl:

➢ 20 lbs x 10 reps

➢ 30 lbs x 8 reps

➢ 40 pounds x 6 reps

- Drop sets are like inverted pyramids with many variations. In one example, it is raised until it fails, regardless of the number of people in the second and third sentences. Start with the heavy ones and do the calculated amount of iterations. Reduce the weight by 20 per cent, for example, and set the next sentence to errors. Then reduce it again and fail again after a short interval. This is a potent workout. An example is a dumbbell curl as follows:

- 40 pounds x 8 reps

- 30 lbs X obstacle

- 20 lb X obstacle

- Super slow. Super Throw encompasses the concept of slow and measured concentric and eccentric contractions. The proposed benefits are controversial. Super slow enthusiasts recommend about 10 seconds for each phase of the lift.

➢ Eccentric training. This emphasizes the return or descending movement of the elevator based on this, which leads to better hypertrophy as more muscle damage and fibre recruitment are achieved. Arm Curl is a good example. Support is usually required to complete the concentric circles or elevators.

➢ Sports-specific programs have been specifically designed to improve the performance of individual sports by strengthening the muscular fitness of those sports through regular strength training.

COMPLETE THE FOUR-WEEK TRAINING

Overview of beginner workouts

➢ Week 1: whole body division

➢ Week 2: divided into two days: upper body / lower body

➢ 3rd week: 3 days divided: push / pull / leg

➢ Week 4: divided into four days: the whole body

WEEK 1: THE ONE

The program begins with a breakdown of the whole body workout. This means training all the important parts of the body in each workout instead of "sharing" the workout. They train for three days in the first week and work only once per body part in each session. It is important to take a day off between each workout to help your body recover. This offers training on Monday, Wednesday and Friday with rest days on Saturday and Sunday.

The exercises noted in Week 1 are a combination of basic movements but are also used for advanced lifters, but I think they are also suitable for beginners. Remember that it's not just about training the device. There will soon be a handful of free weights. The reason for this is these are exercises you need to master for the long-term benefits of muscle size and strength. So you should learn them immediately. Please read all the exercise instructions carefully before trying it yourself.

In the first week, you do three sets of all exercises per workout. This gives up to 9 sets of each body part in a week, making it the first volume that suits your purpose. Repeat 8-12 times per game, without abdominal muscles. This person's regimen is generally considered ideal for achieving increased muscle size (scientific hypertrophy) and is often used by both amateurs and professional bodybuilders.

The following workouts require 8 in the first set, 10 in the second set and 12 in the third set. In bodybuilding circles, this is called the "inverse pyramid" (the standard pyramid moves from higher to lower). Reduce the weight of each set to reach a higher number of employees. For example, if you used £ 140 for eight iterations in the first set of latitude pulldowns, try using £ 120 or £ 130 for Set 2 and £ 100-120 for Set 3.

WEEK 2: SHARED DECISION

It's only a week after the program starts, but you'll use a two-day workout split to work out different parts of your body on different days (i.e., train your entire body in two days instead of the first). Week)). This week we will prepare a total of 4 days. The division includes two upper-body days (Monday and Thursday) and two lower-body days (Tuesday and Friday), and each part of the body is trained twice. Recovery days are Wednesday, Saturday and Sunday.

Some exercises from the first week are carried over to the second week. Still, except for the abdominal muscles, a movement is added to each part of the body routine to train all muscle groups more fully from several angles. You can. For example, the chest contains two exercises. One is a compound movement (weight bench press) that moves the maximum possible number of muscles in multiple joints (both shoulders and elbows), and the other is a separate exercise (barbell fly). It contains only one joint (shoulder) and guides the chest over a larger area. (The deltoids and triceps muscles are somewhat involved in compressing the chest, which means that the pressure force doesn't isolate the chest muscles like a fly.)

Again, we set repetitions in the reverse pyramid scheme, but in the second week, the recurrences (15) in the third sentence of each exercise are slightly higher. Fifteen employees may be outside the ideal muscle-building area, but these sets increase muscle endurance and provide a solid foundation for building future size and strength. Help too.

WEEK 3: THREE APPROACHING

In the third week of the performance, we will do a three-day training split. Exercise all "pressing" parts of the body (chest, shoulders, triceps) on the first day. On the second day, hit the "pulling" parts of the body (back, biceps) and abdominal muscles. On the third day, work on the lower body (quadriceps, gluts, hamstrings, calves). As in the second week, I go to the gym for six days this week to train every part of my body twice a week.

A new exercise has been added to each body part routine that gives you even more angles to train your target muscles and promote full development. Apply 3-3-4 sets of two exercises to each muscle group. Four games of large body parts (chest, back, shoulders, quads, hamstrings) and three sets of small body parts (biceps, triceps, abdomen, calf). As a result, the total weekly collection for large body parts is 16, and the complete set for small pieces is 12. This also works in the range of 8 to 15 repetitions. This is a significant increase in volume from the first week.

WEEK 4: INCREASE THE VOLUME

In the fourth and last week of the program, you will be trained at four-day intervals for four days, with each part of the body being hit only once (calves and abdominal muscles are trained twice). A four-day split is standard for experienced lifters because less body training (typically 2-3) is required per workout. As you can see, the chest and triceps are paired, and the quad with biceps and hamstring is back. Both are prevalent couples between beginners and Advance.

The repetition plans are still bloated this week, but adding sets to individual exercises increases the overall volume. This volume increase ensures that enough muscles are overloaded to continue the growth that started in the first three weeks. After completing this four-week program, you can proceed to the next level.

Ced bodybuilder. The shoulder training is more or less independent and changes with every other training with noticeable calves and abdominal muscles. No new exercises were introduced in week 4, so you can concentrate on your training intensity instead of learning new movements.

STRETCH PROGRAM

Your first goal should be to increase flexibility before starting a fitness program. If you are considering starting a fitness program and have been idle for years, you need to stretch for a week before you start running, doing weight training, or doing gymnastics... You can run to warm up. Therefore, in the first 1-2 weeks after beginning a fitness program, stretch 1-2 times a day, drink 2-3 liters of water a day and go walking, cycling or otherwise have low-intensity aerobic stress with no effect. You have to exercise. 10-15 minutes.

Please follow the stretch table after training. Hold these stretches or make each of these movements for at least 15 to 20 seconds.

➢ Shrug

➢ Chest/biceps stretch

➢ Arm/shoulder stretching

➢ Triceps / backstretch (crescent)

➢ Gastric stretching

➢ Waist stretching

➢ ITB / hip stretching

➢ Stretch the hamstring

➢ Thighs stretching on the floor

Stretching in this order helps to extend the main muscle groups. Widening the connecting groups of the thighs and thighs initially helps to expand the main muscle groups of the body, the ham and the thighs, more completely.

STRETCH AND WARM-UP

The best way to end your workout is to hold these stretches for 15 to 20 seconds. Do not rebound on these stretches, inhale deeply for 3 seconds, hold for 3 seconds and then exhale fully. Do this twice for each route. This takes at least 15 to 20 seconds to keep these stretches for optimal results.

STRETCH DESCRIPTION

ARM / SHOULDER CIRCLE:

Slowly rotate your shoulder in a large circle for 15 seconds. It is like swimming back and front crawl swimming.

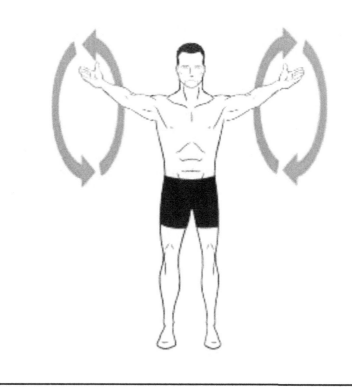

_____

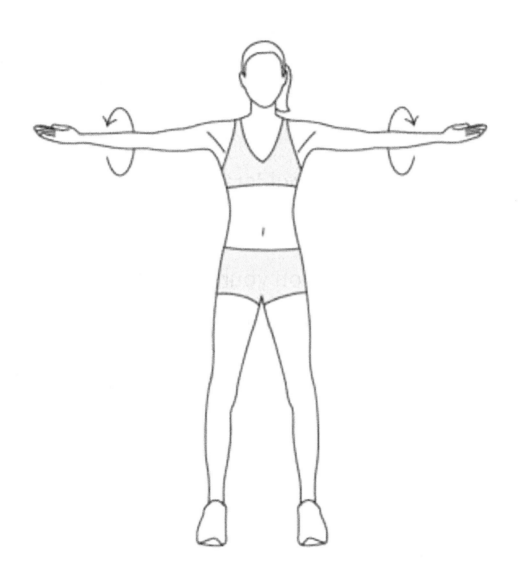

CHEST / SHOULDER / UPPER BACK STRETCH:

Take a bar or wall and twist the opposite side of your arm until you feel a closer connection between your chest and shoulder. Repeat with the other arm. Option 2 Swimmer stretch: keep your hands behind your back, and your shoulders upright with your chest stretched out. Then put your shoulders forward and your chin on your chest. Arm Shoulder Stretch - Grasp your arm with the opposite arm and stretch your back shoulders and upper back to pull it all over your body. Turn your hand with your thumb down.

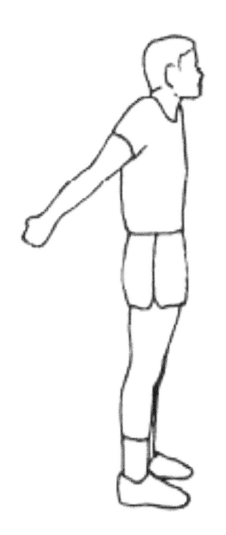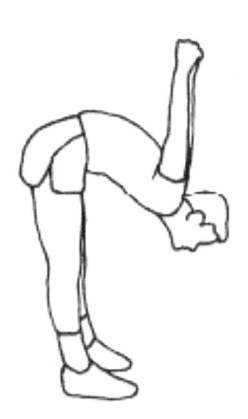

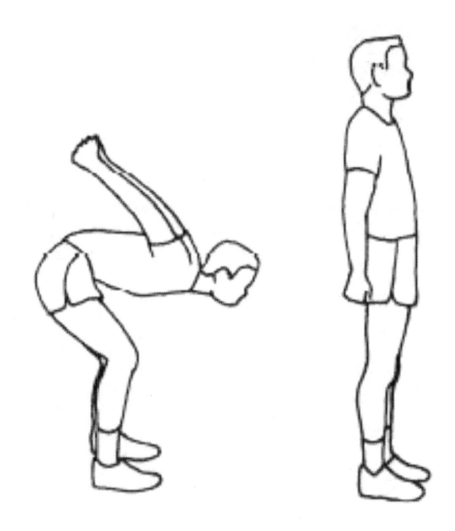

SHOULDER ROTATION:

This movement warms the rotator cuff of the shoulder joint—ideal for throwing the ball or when you need to work over the entire shoulder movement area.

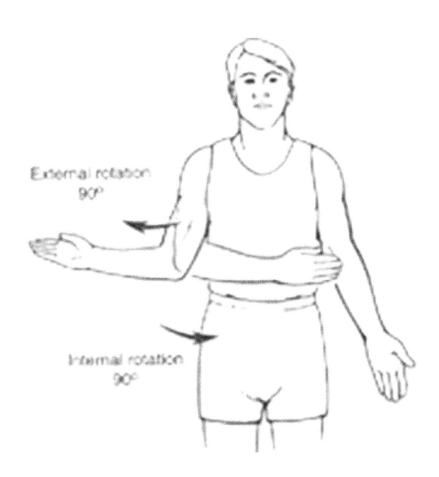

WAIST STRETCH # 1:

Cat Stretch - Bow on all fours as shown. Hold your head as close to your shoulders as possible. Place your chin on your chest and hold it down for 10 seconds.

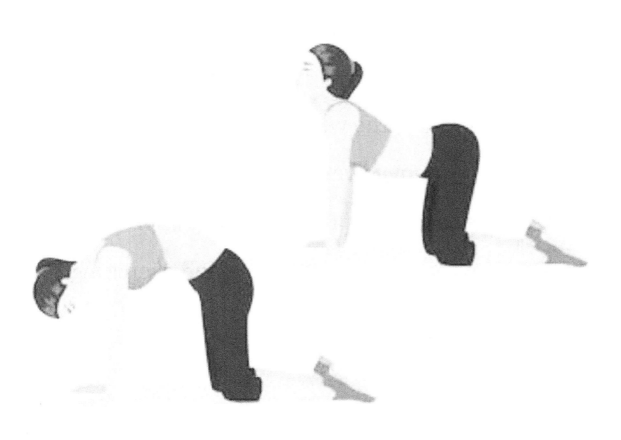

WAIST STRETCH # 2:

is on the left. Place your upper limbs in front of you. Gently twist your torso until your shoulders touch the floor. Hold for 15 seconds and repeat on the right side.

As you may know, the waist is the most commonly injured part. Many lower back problems result from lack of exercise, lack of flexibility, and improper lifting of heavy objects. Stretching and exercising can help prevent injuries.

HIP / THIGH OUTER STRETCH:

Sit with your left leg over your right leg. Grasp the left leg with both hands around the thigh/shin (with the legs bent), pull it towards the chest and then turn it. Repeat with the other leg.

Calf stretch to Achilles tendon stretch stands one foot 2-3 feet in front of the other. Place most of your weight on foot behind you with both feet in the same direction and stretch your calf muscles. Then bend your back knee slightly and should feel the heel stretch. This stretch prevents inflammation of the Achilles tendon. Achilles tendonitis is a severe injury that most people avoid for around 4 to 6 weeks.

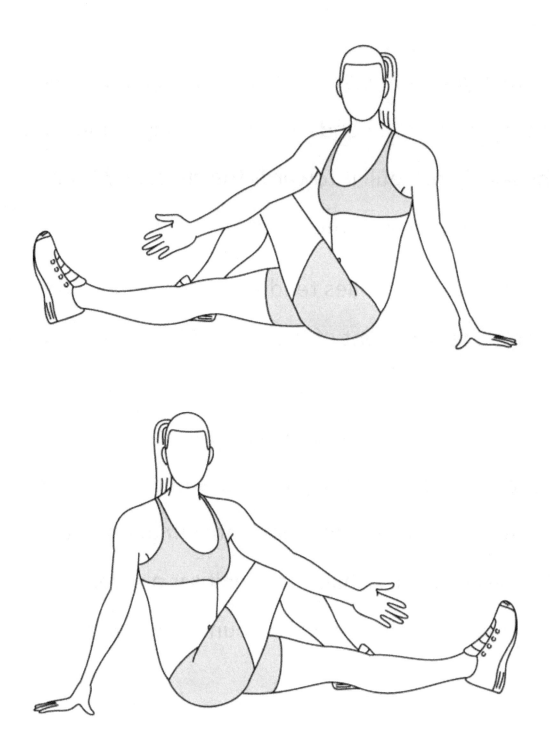

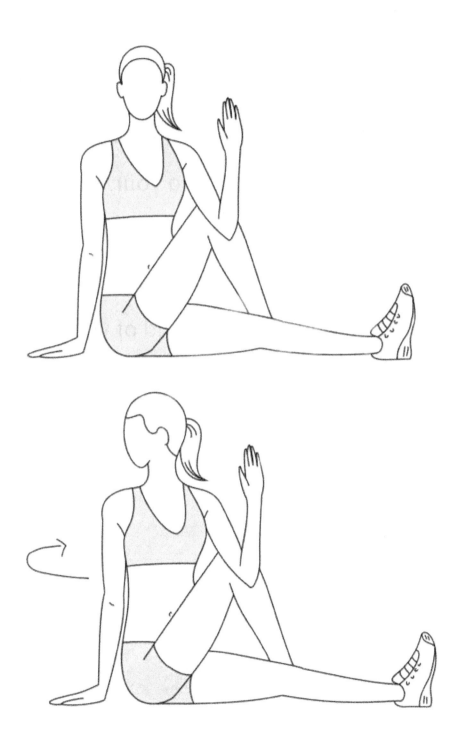

DOWN DOG POSE:

 A relaxed yoga pose that stretches your back and legs. Hold the heel on the floor for 15 to 30 seconds. Knee tendon stretching - Bend your hips forward while standing or sitting and touch your toes. Keep the back straight, then bend the knees slightly. You will feel how you stretch the end of your thigh.

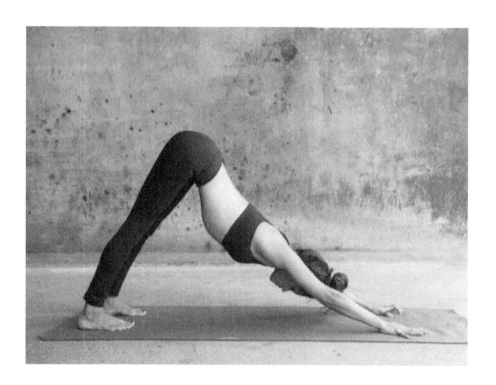

STRETCH THIGH-STAND:

Stand up, bend your knees, and grab your ankles. Pull your heels to your hips and push your hips forward. Squeeze the cheeks of the buttocks and close the knee. Hold the snap-down for 10-15 instants and repeat the process with the other leg (you can keep your balance if necessary or lie on your hips to do this stretch.

Lean, thin exercises: If you get a flat sprint to run or walk, there are two great exercises to build your shin. Stand on your heels for 10-15 seconds. Repeat this numerous times completely the day to build up your shaft. Do 30-40 flex / stretching exercises (2/3 photo) on each leg before walking and running.

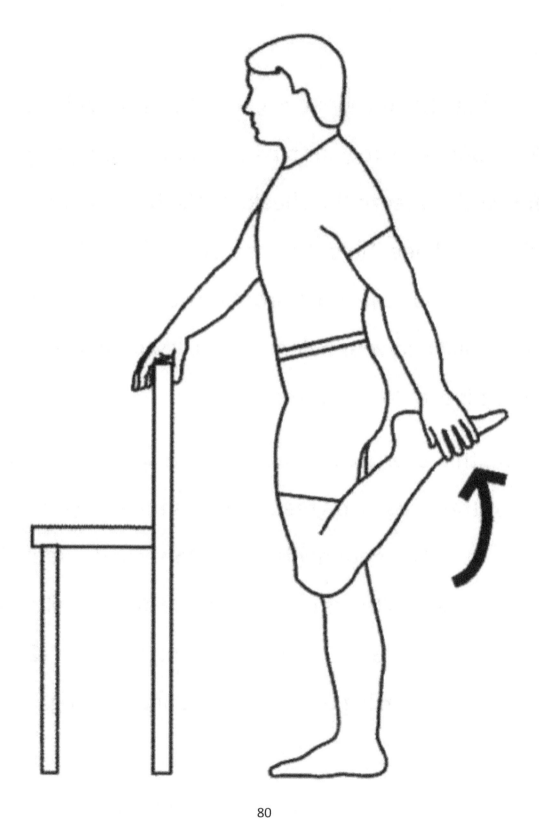

DESCRIPTION

Regular pushups and knee pushups - Lie on the floor next to your chest with your hands. Keep your hands about shoulder-width apart. Extend your arms, stiffen your back and lift your body. In this exercise, you build and secure your shoulders, arms, and chest. Use your knees as needed to complete the training iteration.

Supported Pushups - Use furniture to place your hands 3 to 4 feet above the floor and lean against the furniture or the wall. Keep your arms, back, hips and legs straight and away from well-positioned furniture. Bend your arms so that your chest is in contact with the furniture. Repeat if necessary. This is an excellent place to start if you can't do pushups at all.

Bench dip-sit on a chair, bench or small table. When you sit on the edge of the seat, raise your feet about 3 feet. Then, take the side of the place with your hands and lift your hips off the seat, bend your elbows, and lower them about 4 to 5 inches from the rear.

LOWER BODY EXERCISES

SQUATS:

Spread your legs wide. Lower your hips as if you were sitting in a chair. Concentrate on squeezing your GLUTEs with an upward movement. Keep your heels on the floor and keep your shins almost vertical. Extend your hips back. Do not put your hips on your feet and do not stretch your knees over your feet. This picture is half a crouch - if you can come down without pain, do so.

1/2 SQUATS:

Strengthen your squats by doing 1/2 squats. Hold the pose in a full squat and push yourself up and down within a 6-inch range of motion.

WALK SQUATS:

This is a regular squat but adds a side hop. Squat in a full squat. Mix your feet left or right as you push yourself up. Stop at every step and crouch. If you don't have much space, you can alternate left and right or cross the room for a 10-sided squat to the left and a 10-sided squat to the right to return to your starting point.

right position

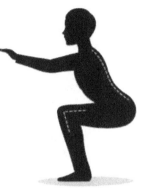
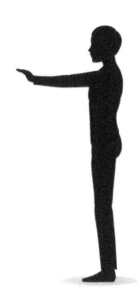

wrong position

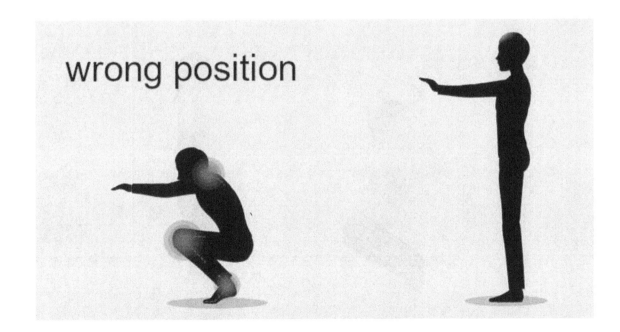

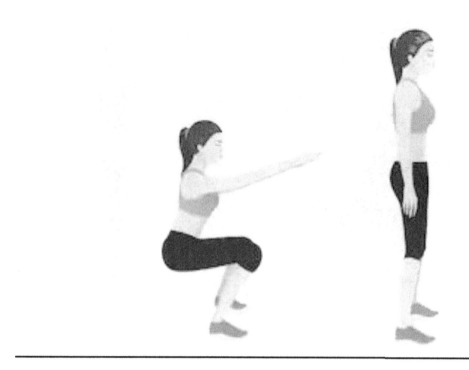

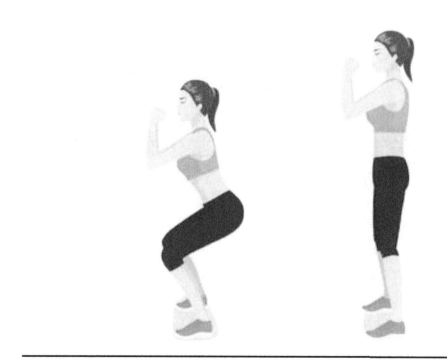

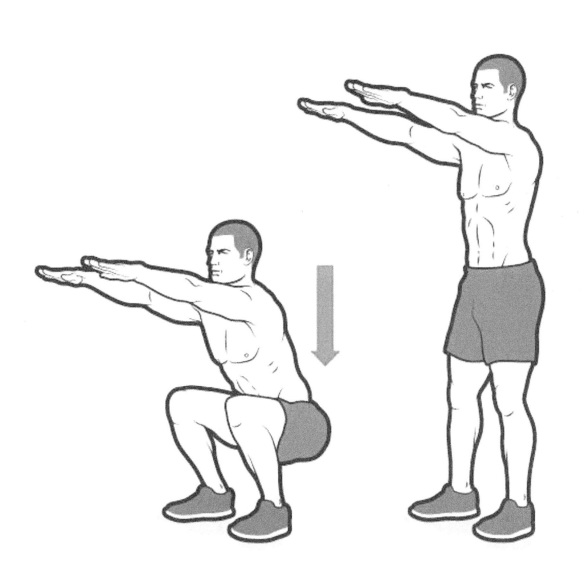

TRAINING DESCRIPTION:

Walking lung lungs are excellent leg exercises for more shape and flexibility. Raise your chest and tense your stomach. Before taking a long step, let your knee drop to the floor.

Stand up with your forefoot, align your feet and repeat with the other foot.

Make sure your knees are not over your feet. In other words, keep your shins vertical. Muscles used: quads, ham, gluts.

STATIONARY LUNGE:

a big step forward. Bend both knees as you lower so that your front legs are parallel to the floor.

Extend your knees but keep your feet in the same position. If you have a bad knee, avoid lunge movements or lower it halfway.

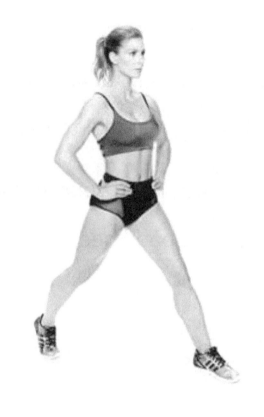

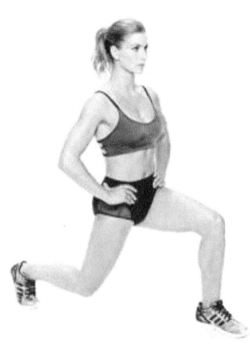

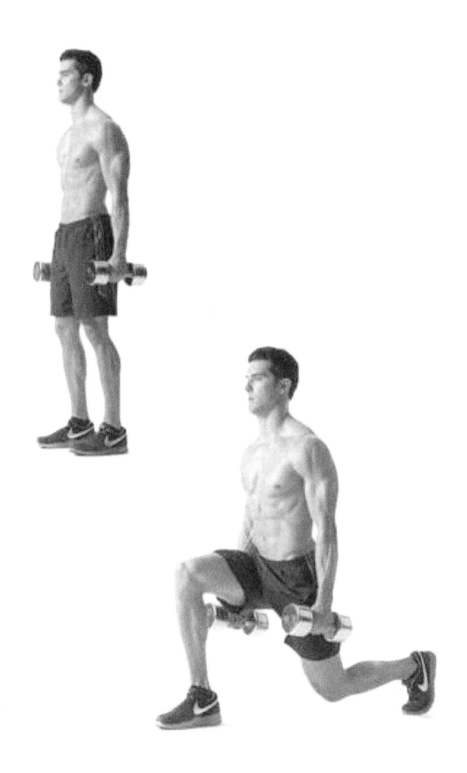

SECTION:

When training your abs, be sure to stretch your back. The abdominal and lumbar muscles are different muscle groups, and if one is much stronger than the other, it can injure a weak muscle group, usually the lower back.

REGULAR CRUNCH:

Lie in the air with your knees bent and feet and knees on your back. Put your hands on your chest, twist your stomach and put your elbows on your knees. If your hips are weak or you were previously injured, keep your feet on the floor.

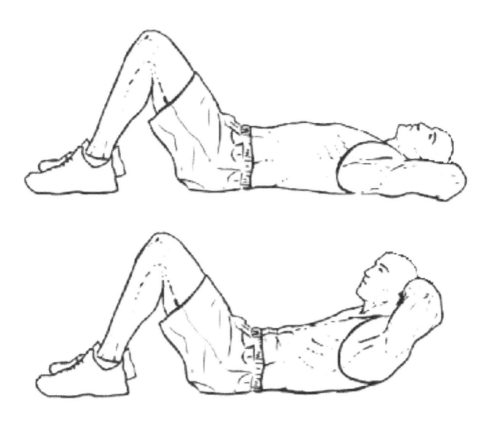

REVERSE CRUNCH:

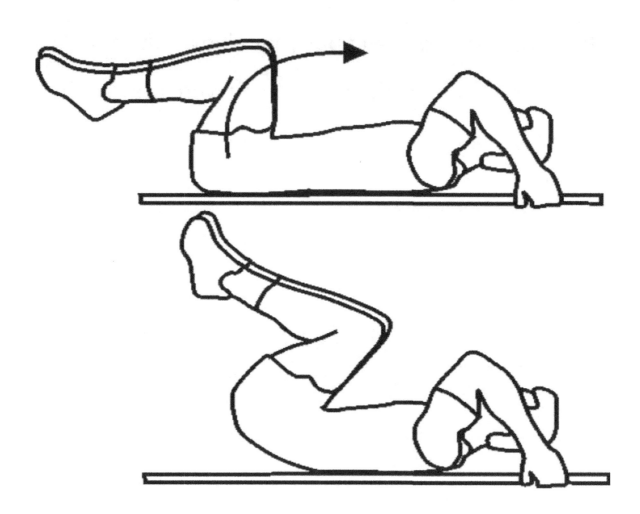

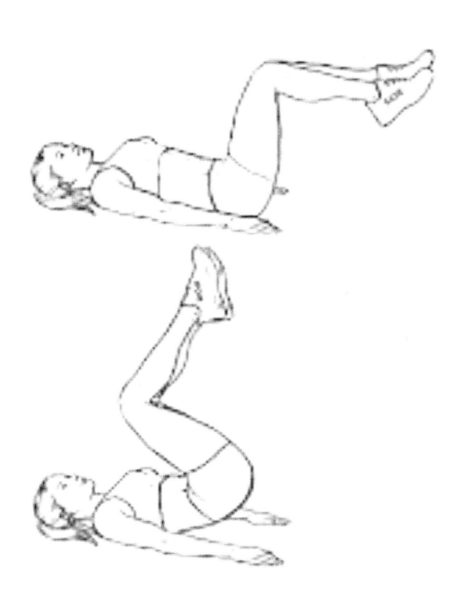

DOUBLE CRUNCH- (LIE LEGS):

Lie on your back with your legs in the air. Bend, bend your belly, put your elbows on your knees and lift your hips like a reverse crunch from the floor. These are two crunches in one go. (Don't do this if you have had a waist injury before

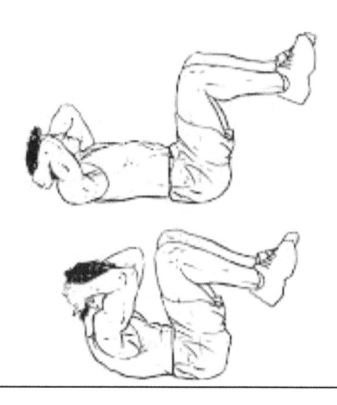

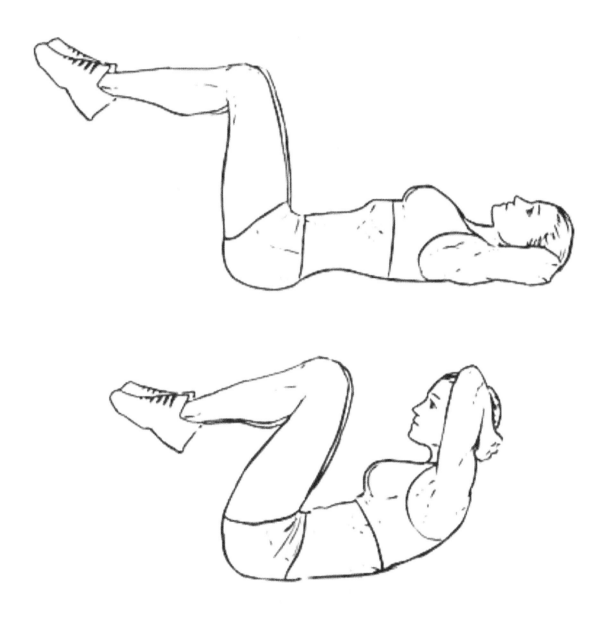

BICYCLE CRUNCH (LOVE GRIPS):

As you grind left and right, move your foot back and forth as shown. It is difficult. So if you have back pain, stop and keep it until your waist is tight.

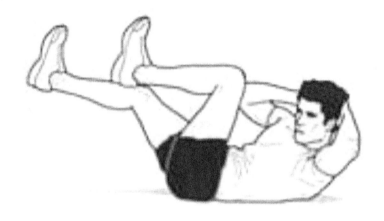

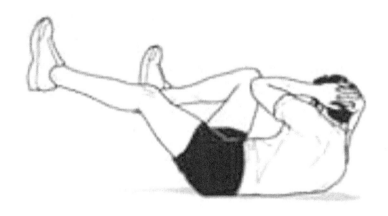

EXERCISE FOR THE UPPER BACK- (REVERSE PUSH UP):

 Lie on your stomach in the Down Push Up position. Instead of pressing on the floor, raise your hand 2-3 inches above the level. This strengthens the upper back muscles, which counteract the pectoral muscles.

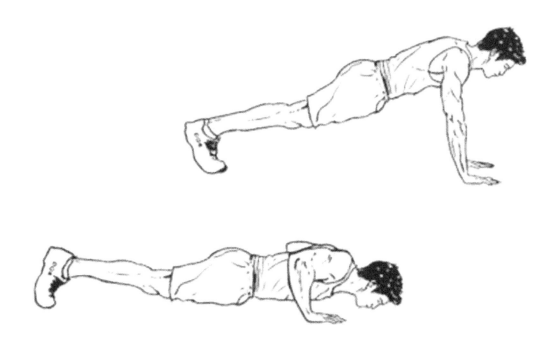

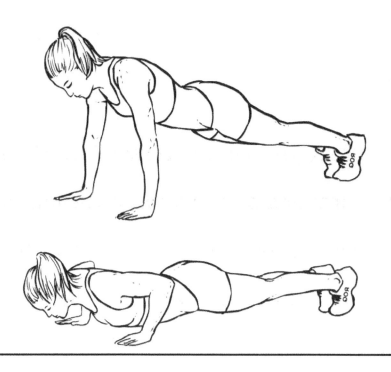

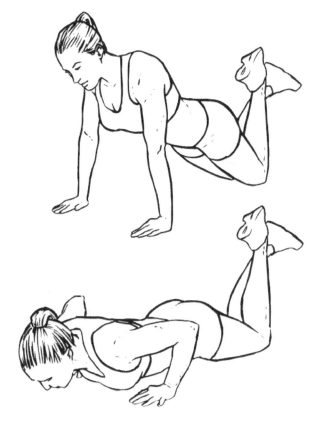

EXERCISE FOR THE UPPER BACK:

Spread your arms at shoulder level and lie on your stomach. Raise your arms from the floor until your shoulder blade "pinches" and slowly put them in the lower position. Imitate the flight of a bird and repeat 10 to 15 times.

LIGHT SHOULDER EXERCISES:

See shoulder exercises in the training table ... See these six exercises...

The following series of exercises are carried out by ten people without interruption.

Side rays-10 (palm)

Side rays - 10 (good)

Side rays-10 (not good enough)

Front rays - 10 (good)

Cross-10 (palm not facing you)

Military press-10

LATERAL RAISE:

Light and weightless, safe and effective shoulder exercise. Dumbbells over 5 pounds are not recommended for this exercise. Bend your knees slightly, hold your shoulders back and hold your chest up. Lift the weight in a smooth, controlled motion parallel to the floor with your palms facing the floor. Follow the next six exercises without stopping.

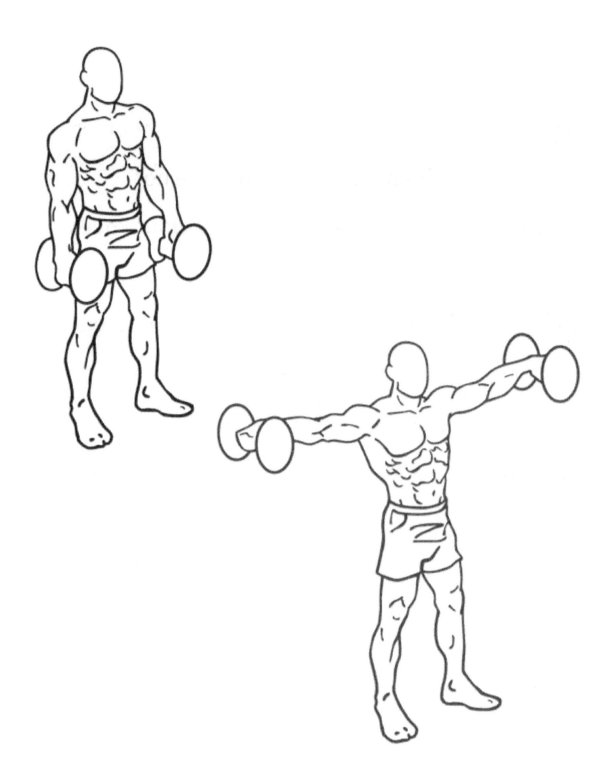

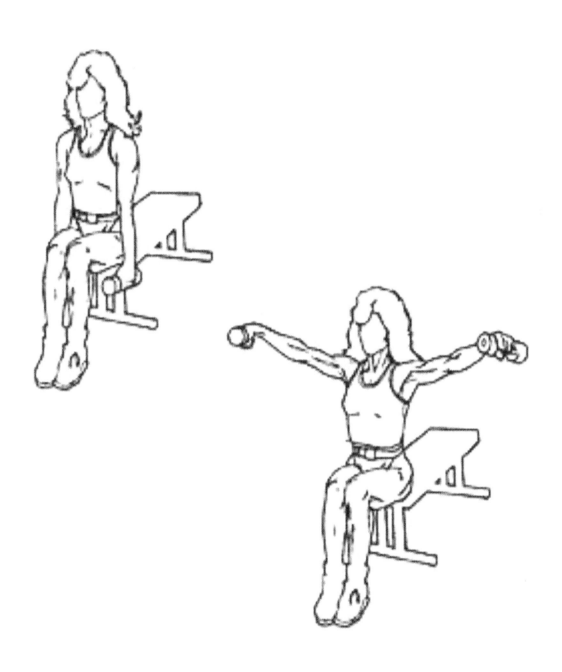

FRONT RAISE (THUMBS UP):

Well, it's time to move the front deltoid muscle by repeating it ten more times. Lift the dumbbells from your waist to shoulder height with your thumb raised.

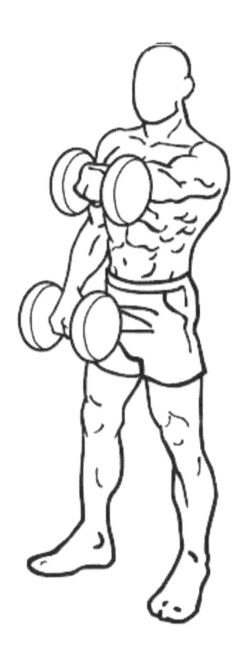
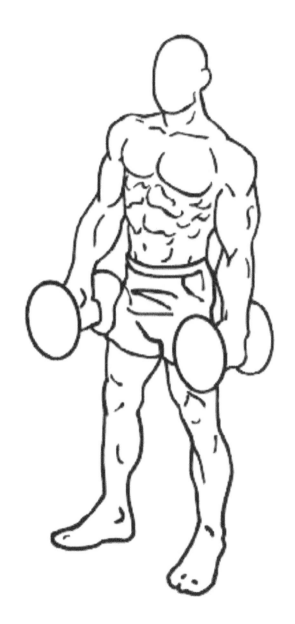

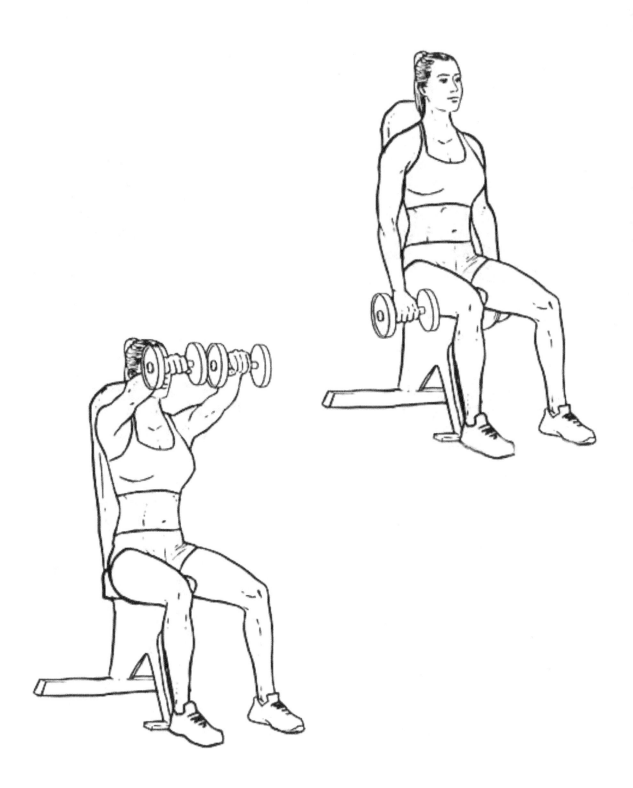

CROSSOVER:

Put, your palms on your back, relax your arms in front of your hips and put your arms over your head as if you were jumping Jacks (without jumping). Cross your arms in front of your head and repeat ten times to get your hips back.

Military press Place one foot in front of you as shown below and bend your knees slightly to reduce the strain on your lower back. Exhale as you push weights over your head in the last ten iterations of the Mega Shoulder Pump Training. Slowly lower to shoulder level and repeat. The muscles used are the shoulder and triceps (back of the arm).

DUMBBELL EXERCISES VARIANTS:

Place the barbell or bar on your hand with the palm of your bicep facing up. Uses the entire range of motion and keeps it smooth. Don't shake the weight—only the elbow moves. Muscles used: biceps (arm).

HAMMER CURL:

Like the upper arm curl, except that the palm is facing the waist. Alternately lift each barbell as you walk - "lips to hip". Uses the entire range of motion and keeps it smooth. Don't shake the weight.

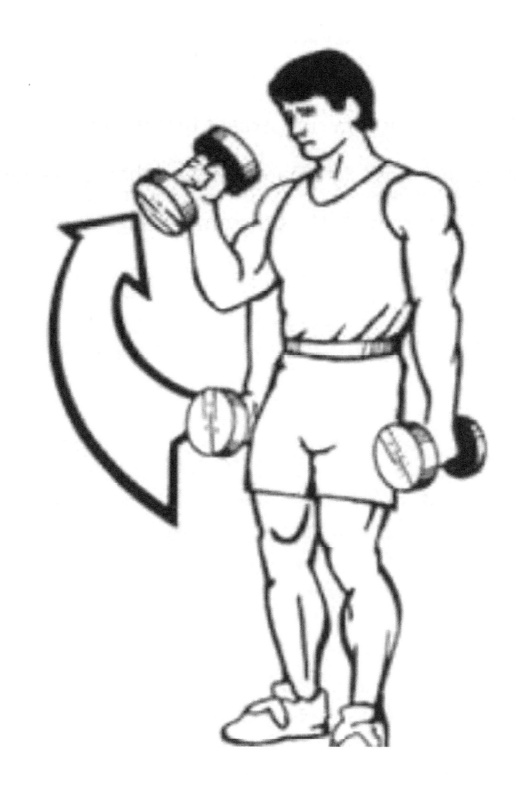

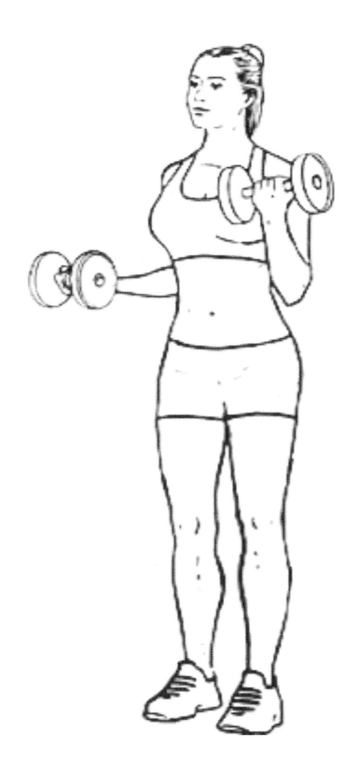

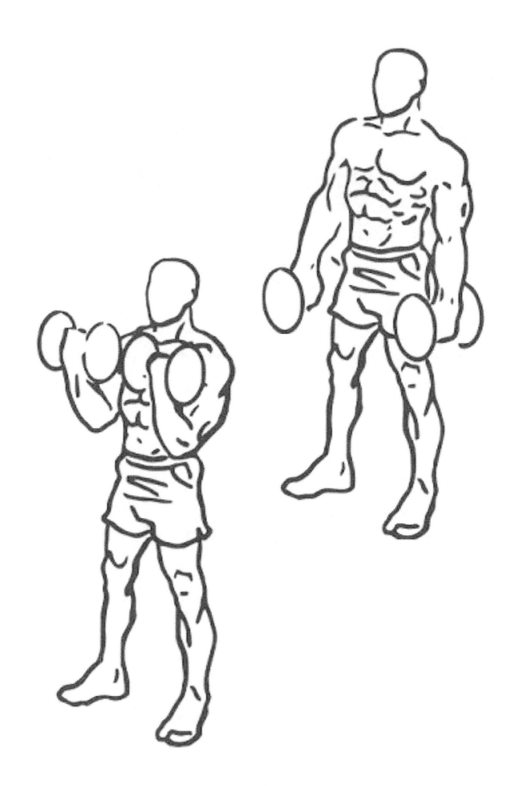

SEATED CURLS:

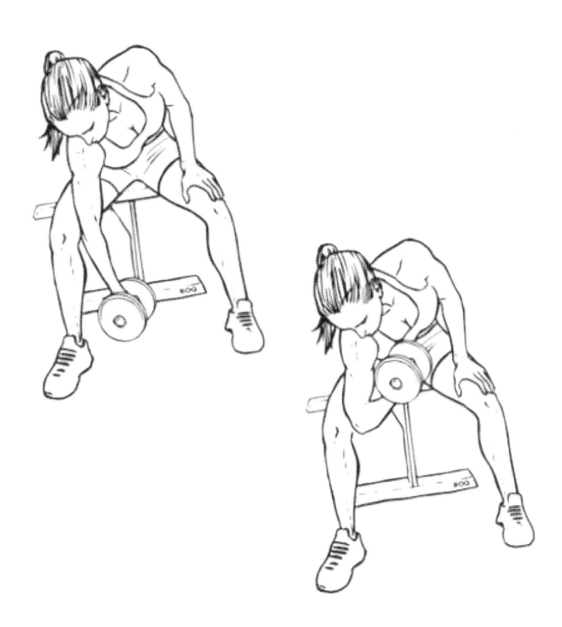

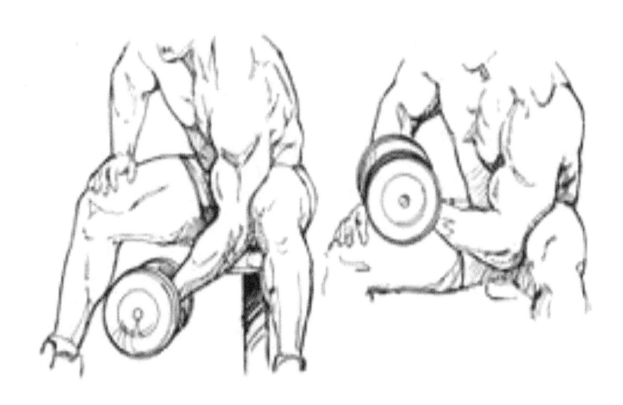

TRICEPS EXTENSION:

Hold the weight (on the back of your arm) in your hand, move your hand over your head, and lower the pressure towards your neck. Move your elbow next to your ear and hold it in place. To repeat!

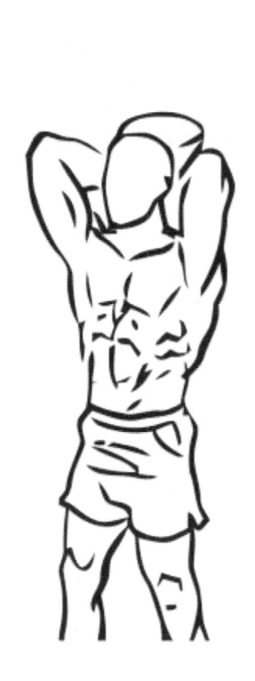
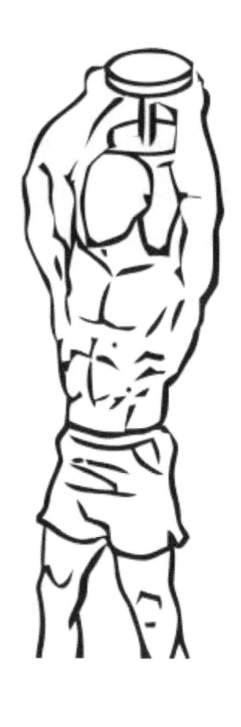

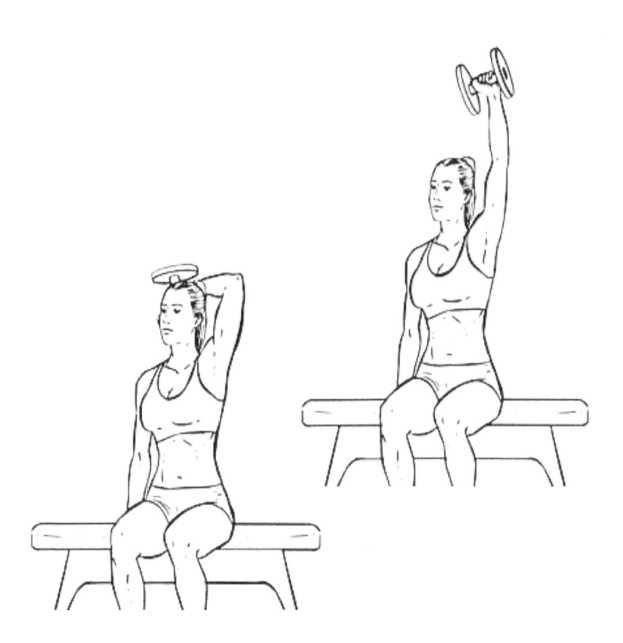

WEIGHT LOSS HELP:

The following pages provide brief instructions on nutrition, hydration, and exercise. We recommend that you continue exercising and stretching next week. Also, note the attached calorie table and how much use you need to "burn out" a particular food. The amount of exercise required can prevent you from eating extra help or a lunch snack during a soccer game.

THINGS TO LEARN AND CARE

EXERCISE AND HEALTH ARE TOP PRIORITIES

The purpose of an exercise program is to reduce fat without losing muscle and without lowering your metabolism. The exercise should be tailored to your specific goals like fitness and fat loss. The combination of cardio and weight training is an ideal combination of exercise to achieve fat loss and should be part of your lifestyle

AEROBICS

Aerobic exercise metabolizes calories and increases metabolism. Your heart rate should be raised to a comfortable level at least three times a week for 20 to 30 minutes. Aerobic exercise consumes more than 300 calories an hour, depending on your weight and fitness.

If you think that only a pound of body fat has about, with 4,100 calories, you can get a rough idea of how long it will take to lose those extra pounds permanently. Look again at the time it took to get dressed, usually a few years, or the entire lifespan of your physical abuse. I recommend working for at least 20 to 30 minutes at a level that you know is sustainable.

The controversy arises when various fitness facilities offer training with a maximum heart rate of maximum 75/90% or light with a maximum heart rate of maximum 55/80% in a short time. I'm going. Put, try both methods. If you are not a complete beginner in fitness, it is best to train as comfortably and as long as possible at a steady pace. Aerobic exercise also increases your metabolism for about 1 minute. Twenty-four hours after the end of the training. This consumes additional calories and prevents a decrease in the metabolic rate.

STRENGTH TRAINING

Inactive people lose about 10% of their muscle mass every ten years after the age of 25. However, regular strength training can regain this muscle mass. Strength training is done 2-3 times a week for about a week. 30 minutes. While weight training is generally not sufficient as an aerobic workout for calories burned, it burns around 250-500 calories an hour, increasing your metabolism. Weight training does not develop your body like bodybuilders, but it does create the ability to burn more calories within 24 hours.

Another critical point is that your muscles do not become fat even after you have finished training.

Muscle tissue naturally breaks down and shrinks. Because lean muscle is more substantial than body fat, your actual weight may not change in the early stages of a new lifestyle plan. Do not worry. You will lose weight, but if not, your total body fat will certainly be a healthy percentage compared to lean muscle.

For this reason, avoid using a scale. If you can't even monitor body fat, measure your body in different places instead—waist, chest, abdomen, thighs. Using clothes is also a great way to measure yourself because with a little time and dedication you will find that the clothes fit you perfectly. At some point, usually two to four weeks, you will lose inches and not lose weight.

HEALTHY EATING

Proper nutrition is essential for fat loss, and focusing on health and wellness foods is much more productive than focusing on reducing fat and rejecting favorite foods. Avoiding salt, fat, sugar, additives, preservatives, processed and refined foods and introducing whole grains should be part of your lifestyle change. By eating more fibre and liquid natural foods (fruits and vegetables), you can eat more and reduce your appetite without gaining weight. Whole foods also have a much higher vitamin and mineral content than regular diets, including processed and refined foods.

Diet is a very negative word - I would like to consider it "weight loss food". The following graphic compares the calorie and expenditure values for different foods or activities. It is essential to understand how much effort is required to burn out a particular food. For example, to burn the calories in a chocolate chip cookie, you have to run hard for at least 20 minutes. Cookies have 110 calories. A person has to walk 20 minutes to burn out this one cookie.

DEHYDRATION

It's easy to develop a dehydrated diet that will lose 10 pounds of water in a few days. Many people are encouraged by these quick results. Dehydration of only a few percents of your body weight can lead to deterioration in physical function. Your body contains more than 75% water, and that percentage needs to stay close to that amount to function correctly. Sweat is not just water, but also salt and electrolytes. These compounds help regulate nerve and muscle function. Without it, the entire system would fail, which could be fatal. Once you stop sweating, no mechanism in the body regulates body temperature, and heatstroke can lead to overheating and death.

Using diuretics and laxatives to remove extra fluid from the digestive system causes the kidneys to work too hard and eventually stop working. In this case, the liver helps (if possible) to excrete waste and prevents the main task of metabolizing fat as a source of energy. In short, you turn off your entire metabolism, and your body desperately tries to stick to the rest of the water and fat. This can cause the opposite desired effect. Your body holds water and grease to survive, and I call this camel mode. This process is a vicious cycle. The real way to burn fat and lose weight is to drink water and exercise. I regularly drink more than a gallon of water, but I often exercise more than 2 hours a day. To see the great results of weight loss, we recommend 2-3 quartz women and 3-4 quarts water a day.

The equation is:

$$\text{Fat loss} = \text{water} + \text{oxygen (from cardiovascular training)}$$

Typical and safe weight loss ranges from 2-3 pounds a week with this formula. Further weight loss You lose weight from water - it will come back as soon as it has left. Avoiding salt, fat, sugar, additives, preservatives, processed and refined foods and introducing whole foods should be part of your lifestyle change. By eating more fibre and liquid natural foods (fruits and vegetables), you can eat more and reduce your appetite without gaining weight. Whole foods also have a much higher vitamin and mineral content than regular diets, including processed and refined foods. Diet is a very negative word - I would like to consider it "weight loss food". Cardio and strength training are the ideal combination of exercise to achieve fat loss and should be part of your lifestyle.

TO AVOID MISTAKES

"Inconsistency," says Wheeler. "Consistently bad plans lead to better results than good, unplanned ones." Repetitions and routines help you learn how your body responds best to exercise and what results in you get. Gives a structure that allows achieving.

Consistency outside the gym is equally important. "Even if we train an hour a day, we still have 23 hours to focus on eating, hydrating, and sleeping," says Wheeler.

After all, inexperienced lifters often swing the weights around, causing the weight plate to bounce off the weight stack of the machine. Why? Perhaps it makes them more convenient because you can lift heavy things and show that you are doing well yourself. Experienced lifters maintain tension in the target muscles throughout the focus and focus on contraction and extension.

THIS WAY YOU AVOID (ALSO) DAMAGE

If you have previously done strength training, you may experience late onset muscle pain. DOMS is a pain phenomenon that occurs 12 to 48 hours after exercise, usually after an unknown exercise. It did no irreversible damage. A study published in the Strength and Conditioning Journal entitled "Microscopic connective tissue tears" makes strength experts Brad Schoenfeld and Bret Contreras much more likely. Along with mechanical tension and metabolic stress, it is one of the critical mechanisms in hypertrophy, an increase in muscle size.

You don't have to struggle to grow, but people can develop a joy/pain addiction that has the (harmless) feeling that they won't do enough without pain. "The wildest DOMS is usually highly mobile personnel with a large eccentric or descending phase for hamstrings and GLUTE like deadlifts and lunges in Romania," says Hamilton. You can slow down your trauma by gradually adjusting your weight and staff, or progressively increasing your workload. Secondly, active post-workout recovery promotes muscle repair, increases blood flow, and provides the muscles with oxygen and nutrients. For example, after lunchtime leg training, try not to get stiff with Hamilton's simple solution. When I started catching, I always got an emergency code.

ADVANTAGES OF WEIGHT LIFTING

Strength training isn't just about enlarging your biceps, and it's a welcome bonus. It helps your health in every way. "It stimulates muscle growth, bone strengthening and fat loss," says Dan Trainer, a personal trainer. His iron commitment won his cover of Men's Fitness Australia in 2013.

For this reason, the NHS (not on men's fitness coverage, but worth listening to) ensures that every adult participates in strength training more than once a week and applies to all major muscle groups. Recommended. This is particularly significant as you get older. A durable frame helps to avoid joint and bone problems.

Besides, we should not underestimate the psychological benefits of all types of exercises, and you will find that you can clean your head by spending time in the weight room every week.

"For me, it's a form of meditation," says Wheeler. "It can lead to daily results, both physically and mentally, every time you complete a set or workout."

In this case, weight lifting has countless advantages. It is worth thinking about the unique features that you want to achieve in your training. Recognizing the primary goal of taking up dumbbells motivates you to continue this consistently.

ESSENTIAL WEIGHTLIFTING MOVEMENTS FOR BEGINNERS:

The weight room can feel intimidating when you are new to strength training. Regardless of whether you are completely confused, which weights to use for which exercise, or whether you want to distort your body to fit your machine, there are many uncertainties.

This gymnastics may be very realistic, but getting the most out of it means missing out on all the benefits of weight lifting.

Exercising your muscles not only makes you stronger, but it also increases your confidence and self-esteem when you see what your own body can do. Moving the focus from the weight on the scale to the weight you have in your hand gives you strength. Weight training keeps your bones healthy, and research has shown that it can have other health benefits, such as B. reducing anxiety and improving heart health. I'm going. You will make yourself a real misfortune by letting fear prevent you from taking full advantage.

As a beginner, the best approach to weight lifting is to start with a combination of functional exercises that mimic everyday movements and compound exercises, which are exercises that involve several large muscle groups at the same time. Most functional activities fall into one of the categories squat, push, pull, hip joint, or hip extension. Learning these movement patterns is key to creating the foundation on which you can build more complex exercises.

Exercise is excellent for beginners. Because these exercises start in this practical way, if you master them, you can get used to lifting and be ready to be safe when you get stronger.

If you're starting, choose a weight that you can lift 10 to 12 times in a few sets. This is usually 5 to 15 pounds depending on the muscle group (you can probably use heavier weight on the lower body compared to the upper body). If you are a beginner, you will find that it is time to move over these weights quickly if you feel that the last few reps can be easily increased.

If you have never participated in the Goblet Squat, Romanian Deadlift or Grootbridge weight versions, you will first learn any weight without weight. Using weight alone can help establish the correct technique and shape and reduce the risk of injury before adding weight to the mix. To feel comfortable when lifting the dumbbells, it is recommended to practice these movements 2-3 times a week.

ESSENTIAL WEIGHTLIFTING MOVES FOR BEGINNERS:

GOBLET SQUATS

➢ Place your weight on the chest with hands, your elbows close to the body and your legs a little more scattered than your hips.

➢ Bend your knees and lower your hips into a crouch. Hold your chest up and tighten the core.

➢ Push your knees out to hold the heel weight.

➢ Squeeze the heel to stand up and squeeze the upper part of the buttocks. It is a person.

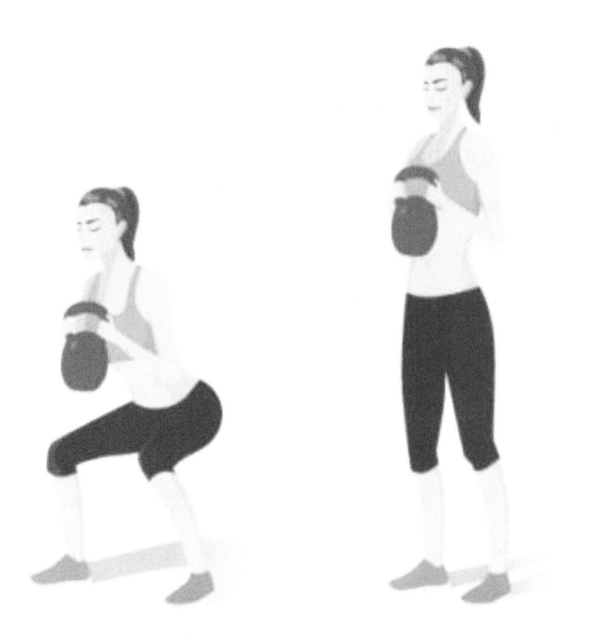

SHOULDER PRESS

➢ Stand with slightly wider legs than your hips or keep your back straight and firm on your knees (see illustration above). With a dumbbell, raise your arms to shoulder level and bend your elbows so that the weights float in the air. Twist the wrist so that your palm is confronting you.

➢ Push the barbell over your head. The elbow should point forward during the press.

➢ Stop the upper part when your arms are fully extended. Then slowly bring the weight back to the starting position. It is a person.

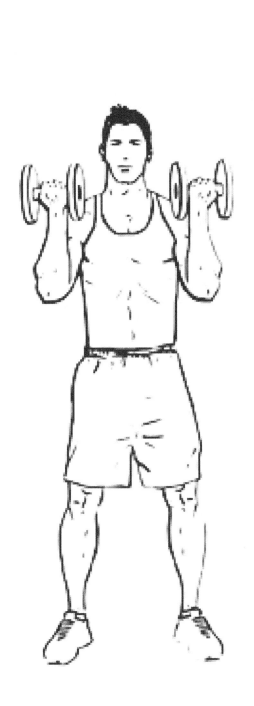
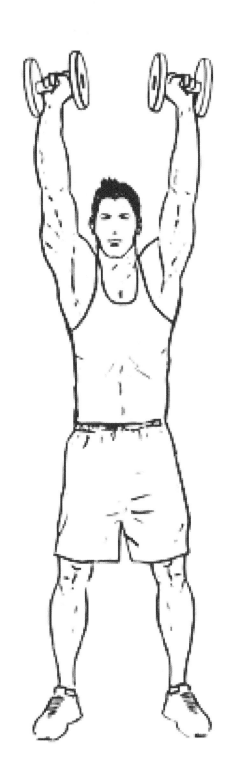

BASIC DEADLIFT DEAD LEG

➢ Hold the dumbbells on both feet, spread your legs over your hips and bend your knees slightly to stand.

➢ Hang your hips and bend your knees slightly when lowering. Push your butt back.

➢ Hold the barbell close to your foot when descending. Do not pull the shoulder blade back and the back should be arched.

➢ Hold your core and push it straight through your heels. Place the weight near the shin as you pull.

➢ Stop at the top and squeeze your hips to complete a person.

CURVED ROW

➤ Hold the barbell with one hand. Put your opposite leg forward and stand in a staggered position. Turn your hips forward, your torso on the floor and your back flat.

➤ Hold your body in this position, raise the dumbbells at chest height and put your elbows aside.

➤ Ground the barbell back toward those starting position in a controlled movement. It is a person.

CHEST PRESS

➢ Recline on the floor or a horizontal bench with the dumbbells in your hands on your back.

➢ Turn your wrist forward so that your palm is facing away from you.

➢ Hold the dumbbells on both contestants of your chest and bend your elbows at a 90-degree angle.

➢ Push the dumbbells together. Use the chest muscles to initiate movement.

➢ Return your arm to its original position. It is a person.

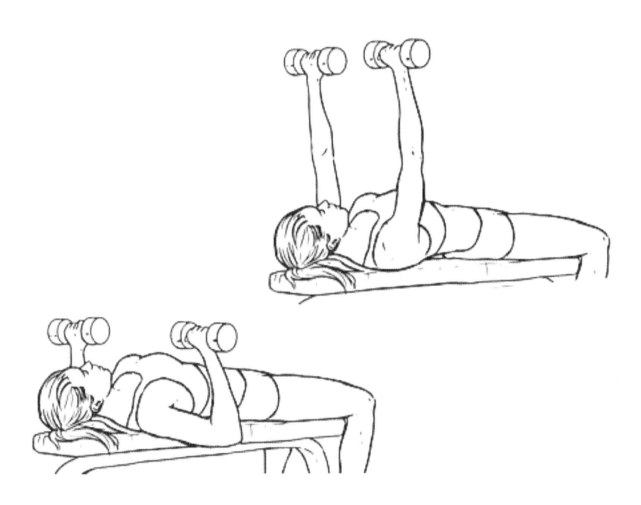

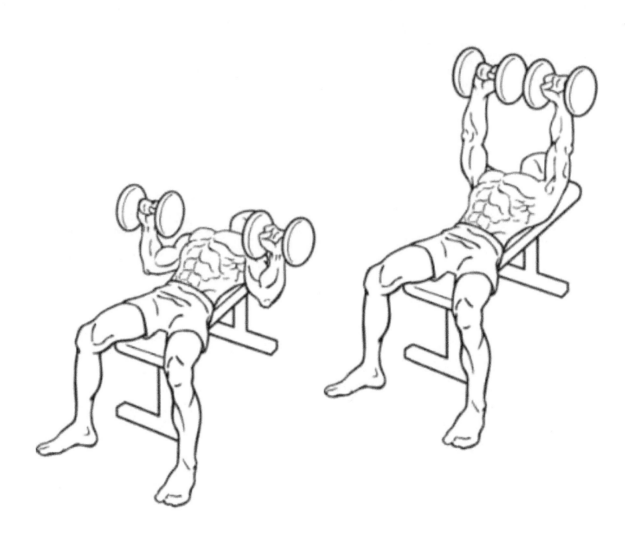

GLUTE BRIDGE

➢ Bend your knees, feet on the floor, dumbbells on your hips and your back. Keep your heels a few inches from your buttocks, and your feet should be about from your bones.

➢ Squeeze the glute and press on your heels to raise your lower back. Make a diagonal line from the shoulder to the knee.

➢ Stop for 1-2 seconds and then slowly lower yourself to the floor. It is a person.

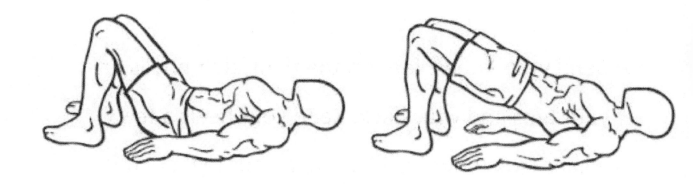

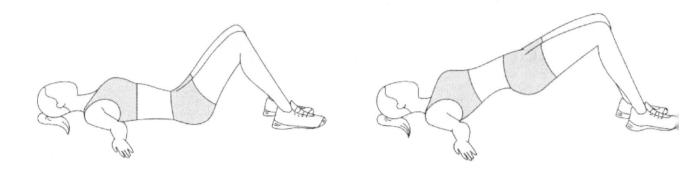

PUSH-UPS

Check your push-ups slowly. Lower 2 seconds and return 2 seconds. After putting up one of the push-ups, press your back on the floor.

CHEST PRESS

Lie on the floor with your back, lift the barbell and push it towards the ceiling. Slowly focus on your pectoral muscles and what you are doing. Let us rest for 2 minutes and run the next push-up press set.

SQUATS

Start without leaning. Use dumbbells when you get used to it. Push your hips back while squatting to avoid putting pressure on your knees.

DEADLIFT

Drive straight from one of the squats to heavy lifting. Keep control of your body and go slowly. After resting for 2 minutes, go back and do the other two combo sets.

PULLING UP

This is one of the most challenging exercises for beginners. Please do as much as you can. If you need help, move up with a band or chair, slowly step back and repeat the process. Go straight to the line after the first sentence.

LINE

When using dumbbells, bend the rows. If you are using a band, please sit in a row. You are slowly in control as you benefit most from your efforts.

CURL

Go slowly with dumbbells and ribbons. Keep your elbows aside and don't use the momentum to help curls. Go to the triceps cave immediately after the set.

DIP

Dip your hands behind your back on your chair or bench. Start by putting your foot on the floor. As you get stronger, put your feet on the chair and add resistance.

SHOULDER PRESS

You can do this while sitting or standing. Hold the barbell at shoulder height and slide it over your head. Do the same if you use ribbons.

PLANK

Move to a push-up position on your elbows instead of your hands, stretch your body, and hold that position for 30 seconds for each person. Let it rest for 15 seconds and contact another person. Run five people, and you're done.

Kind reader,

Thank you very much. I hope you enjoyed the book.

Can I ask you a big favor?

I would be grateful if you would please take a few minutes to leave me a gold star on Amazon.

Thank you again for your support.

John McDillon

Made in the USA
Las Vegas, NV
21 December 2023

83339896R00090